Oil Pulling Beginner's Guide!

Oil Pulling

I0420053

Learn How To Heal Your Body Using Nature's Ancient Detoxifying And Healing Oil Pulling Oral Detox Therapy Cleansing!

Sarah Brooks

Copyright © 2015 Sarah Brooks

STOP!!! Before you read any further....Would you like to know the secrets of Anti-Aging?

If your answer is yes, then you are not alone. Thousands of people are looking for the secret to reducing wrinkles, looking younger, and maintaining a youthful appearance.

If you have been searching for these answers without much luck, you are in the right place!

Not only will you gain incredible insight in this book, but because I want to make sure to give you as much value as possible, right now for a limited time you can get full **100% FREE access to a VIP bonus EBook** entitled **Anti-Aging Made Easy!**

<u>**Just Go Here For Free Instant Access:**</u>

<u>**www.LuxyLifeNaturals.com**</u>

Legal Notice

All rights reserved. Without limiting the rights under the copyright reserved above, no part of this publication may be reproduced, stored in or introduced into a retrieval system, or transmitted, in any form, or by any means (electronic, mechanical, photocopying, recording, or otherwise) without the prior written permission of the copyright owner and publisher of this book. This book is copyright protected. This is for your personal use only. You cannot amend, distribute, sell, use, quote or paraphrase any part or the content within this eBook without the consent of the author or copyright owner. Legal action will be pursued if this is breached.

Disclaimer Notice

Please note the information contained within this document is for educational and entertainment purposes only. Considerable energy and every attempt has been made to provide the most up to date, accurate, relative, reliable, and complete information, but the reader is strongly encouraged to seek professional advice prior to using any of this information contained in this book. The reader understands they are reading and using this information contained herein at their own risk, and in no way will the author, publisher, or any affiliates be held responsible for any damages whatsoever. No warranties of any kind are expressed or implied. Readers acknowledge that the author is not engaging in the rendering of legal, financial, medical, or any other professional advice. By reading this document, the reader agrees that under no circumstances is the author, publisher, or anyone else affiliated with the production, distribution, sale, or any other element of this book responsible for any losses, direct or indirect, which are incurred as a result of the use of information contained within this document, including, but not limited to, -errors, omissions, or inaccuracies. Because of the rate with which conditions change, the author and publisher reserve the right to alter and update the information contained herein on the new conditions whenever they see applicable.

Table Of Contents

Introduction

I want to thank you and congratulate you for purchasing the book, *"Oil Pulling: Oil Pulling Beginner's Guide! - Learn How To Heal Your Body Using Nature's Ancient Detoxifying And Healing Oil Pulling Oral Detox Therapy Cleansing!"*.

This "Oil Pulling" book contains proven steps and strategies on how to make use of the ancient art of oil pulling as a way to achieve better oral health. Yes, you are going to be introduced to a way of treating oral health problems that is seemingly complicated but will turn out to be simple as we explore it.

As an individual who is a part of a fast-paced modern world, you are aware of the fact that maintaining good oral health is very important but difficult at the same time. It is connected to the health of the entire body which is composed of multiple systems that are responsible for vital physiological processes.

With the current health trend of "going back to nature" and the use of all-natural materials, the reintroduction of oil pulling into the limelight is very timely. Yes, you will be using materials (in their unrefined and cold-pressed state) that are deemed safe to the human body.

This book will take you on a learning journey that involves the basics of oil pulling, options for materials, establishing of routines, do's and don'ts, and the advanced or most effective techniques. You don't need to have a background in Ayurvedic medicine to understand the information presented here. Everything has been simplified for you.

Remember to keep an open mind and have the motivation to really explore something that could benefit you a lot in the end.

Thanks again for purchasing this book, I hope you enjoy it!

Chapter 1: What Is Oil Pulling?

Most probably, you have heard already about this thing called as oil pulling. It is actually an innovative way of getting traditional and modern systems of body care and therapy together. If you see people practicing this oil pulling thing, you will notice that they have whiter teeth, fresher breath, and are generally healthy. Those who are practicing it are referring to it as a form of holistic dental care routine.

Oil is basically squished around the mouth and functions as a mouthwash. It is proven to be a good solution for those who are having problems with their dental health. This routine has beneficial effects for the teeth, gums, and of course the entire body. The oil acts as an antibacterial agent, breath freshener, and a booster of immunity.

Before we move on, let us focus on some trivia about the human mouth and the bacteria that are naturally present in it. Yes, you have millions of bacteria in your mouth which is a natural thing because it is the passageway of materials coming from the outside. Make no mistake about this but the right level of bacteria that enters your digestive system is good. It aids in digestion as well as in the excretion of wastes. Problems arise when the delicate balance between good and bad bacteria is disrupted. It all starts in the mouth of course.

Oil pulling requires the use of very specific materials. Many of those who have done it recommend the use of sesame and coconut oil. This is, of course, because of the taste factor. Other types of oil could be used depending on your preferences. The most commonly used out there include peppermint, sunflower, and oregano oil. A tablespoon of oil is squished in the mouth and retained there for at least 20 minutes. This is a long time for many of us but the technique here is to do other tasks while you are oil pulling for the duration of the session.

This is basically done in the morning where the bacterial content in our mouth is highest. It works effectively because when you mix oil and oil (from the cell membrane of bacteria) together, they tend to stick. Oil pulling basically takes out the bacteria that are present in your mouth. The body has its healthy dose of gastrointestinal bacteria. When the level reaches its peak, the body's immunity system will have to work harder. When there is less bacteria to fight off, the immunity system is basically put to work on other systems of the body.

Oil pulling is an age old but very effective way to promote body healing in a natural way. It is mentioned even in ancient medical literature. It could be used as a beauty routine, a hygienic practice, or just a simple way to promote better overall body health. The whole process is simple, cheap, and effective.

Chapter 2: What To Expect And Why It Is Important

Since it is an unusual biomedical procedure, it is a sure thing that oil pulling has been getting into the curious side of your mind. It is common for such types of controversial procedures to have some unique and wild features. Of course, you know that you need to be rational and look at all its aspects before believing any of those outrageous yet impressive claims about oil pulling being posted online these days. You need to have the correct expectations about the whole thing if you are going to try it.

Let us get started on the requirements for oil pulling. Actually, the beauty in this procedure is seen on its simplicity. There are no costly materials needed and no complicated combinations of chemicals to figure out. If a certain company or program requires you to buy a lot of things for the process, then you are probably being scammed.

Yes, you will have to deal with the uncomfortable feeling of having oil in your mouth for 20 minutes. The oil is supposed to be kept moving in the mouth. Squishing is the proper term for the action of moving the oil around the teeth and gums. Expect that the taste will not be that good, most especially if you have not chosen the right type of oil to use. Oregano oil, as an example, is very good when you need its antiseptic properties but it can produce a bit of a spicy sensation on the mouth.

Expect no side effects as the materials used are all natural. There are no restrictions as to who can do oil pulling. The elderly, children, and even pregnant women can do this procedure safely. Oil pulling is best done when you are on an empty stomach.

On a very realistic point of view, you will experience some body reactions that indicate the procedure is really working. There could be a loosening of phlegm in your throat and this comes up the mouth. There is a possibility that the salivation reflex in your mouth could get reduced when you are doing the procedure. This could lead to the oil remaining thick in consistency even after being squished in your mouth for the entire 20 minutes.

Now, why is oil squishing important? Actually, the list of benefits is long and this is what makes it attractive for those who are looking for health and wellness solutions. The way that oil squishing works is very basic but impressive.

Oil pulling is used to cure a wide range of systemic and oral diseases. These include diabetes, ischemic heart disease, fatty liver, and a wide assortment of renal, respiratory, digestive system diseases. The mode of action against chronic and acute diseases will vary. Those who have acute diseases will see improvements after a day or two. Those who have chronic diseases can expect the effects to get manifested for a longer period of time. There are factors that can affect the rate of healing and these include age, nature of disease, and the kind of lifestyle that you have.

Oil pulling is very important because of the fact that it is a simple remedy for health and wellness problems. It doesn't stain the teeth, doesn't leave behind an undesirable smell in the mouth, and it doesn't trigger any form of allergy. By giving you a better level of oral health, the health of all your body's systems are also benefited.

Chapter 3: Best Types Of Oil To Use

If you are already convinced that you are going to try oil pulling, there is one question that would most likely be on your mind. This is all about the kind or type of oil that you are supposed to use for the procedure. Actually, there is no single answer for this question. The options that you have are quite numerous and the choices you will make will depend upon many personal factors.

If we will trace back the Ayurveda principles from which oil pulling is based, the recommendation will be on the use of sunflower oil. However, due to issues of accessibility and availability, sesame seed oil has gained greater popularity a couple of years back. This is the reason why a lot of online guides and articles on oil pulling can be noted unanimously pointing out the use of this material.

If modern biochemical and physiological principles will be considered, coconut oil will be the best one to make use of. The level of Omega-6 oils on this material doesn't disrupt the healthy 3:6 Omega ratio in our body. It is also a type of oil that many of us are exposed to commonly at the current times. We are very familiar with its taste which is pleasant and soothing.

Coconut oil also has antiseptic and antiviral properties. This will increase the effectiveness of the oil pulling procedure that you will do if you will use it. The detoxifying property of coconut oil is also something that has been proven by many researchers.

Actually, the final choice that people will make will depend upon the factor of palatability or taste. Sesame oil has a warming effect. Coconut and sunflower oil have lower energy outputs. Of course, it will be up to you to try which one will be within your comfort zone and actual needs.

It will be better if you can stick to the use of unrefined, organic, and cold-pressed oils. This is because the energy on these types of oil hasn't yet been put off balance. These oils should not have chemical residues if the extraction process is done according to Ayurveda principles. If you'd have trouble getting your hands on unrefined types of oils, coconut and sesame oil could be a good starting point.

Toasted oil is not recommended because the heating process that produced it may have altered its chemical composition. Grape seed oil is another one that might sound good to use but is generally not recommended if you will stick to your goal of going all-organic.

There are people who would mix essential oils and taste improvement additives to the oil used in oil pulling. Doing so may be good for those who are just beginners on the procedure but is not at all recommended. The natural properties and chemical balance of the oil that we are using should not be altered if we're aiming for the best possible results.

Chapter 4: How Oil Pulling Cures Common Oral Problems

As stated in the previous chapters of this book, oil pulling is beneficial for your overall oral health. Take note that oil pulling is not based on pseudo-science. Even if it has ancient origins, its mechanism has been revealed and can be explained by science. Yes, there are studies that have been conducted for the sole purpose of proving that oil pulling really works.

Since it is the mouth where the procedure is done, this is where the benefits can be seen first. Oral problems such as bad breath, gum infections, and other similar conditions have been seen solved by oil pulling routines. This is good news for those who want to take the "organic and natural" way of living.

Now, let us go deeper on the mechanism of oil pulling. How does it work against oral problems? Let us get started by pointing out the natural presence of common bacteria in the mouth. Yes, we are talking about the streptococcus strain. Its plaque and bad breath forming variety, the Streptococcus mutans, could reproduce quickly inside the mouth most especially if you don't have good oral hygiene.

The full mechanism of oil pulling is actually still under research. However, there are already two scientific explanations that we could rely on. These are as follows:

- **Prevention of bacterial product adhesion** – The oil being squished all over the mouth is viscous enough to make the surfaces resistant to plaque adhesion and aggregation. It will also reduce the possibility of bacteria sticking to the surfaces in the inner mouth.
- **Triggering of saponification** – Yes, this is soap-making happening right in our mouth. Oils like sesame oil are made up of vegetable fat. When this reacts with the saliva which contains bicarbonates, the process of saponification

is triggered. The resulting compound is similar to soap which has an emulsifying (fat-breaking) power. This has the capability to cleanse surfaces. Bacteria and bacterial products can then be easily flushed out.

If you will use sesame oil, you can benefit from two unsaponifiable components within it. These include sesamin and sesamolin which form thin and almost unnoticeable protective layers on the surfaces inside the mouth. This action is enough for the prevention of oral infections and other conditions that are linked to it.

Of course, oil pulling doesn't work only on bacteria but also on a wide range of microorganisms that might enter our mouth and cause diseases. Oil pulling has been proven to work against certain species of yeasts, viruses, and even protozoa. This is, of course, a big factor for the effectiveness of oil pulling in maintaining the health of an individual and in the prevention of diseases that are caused by entry of microorganisms through the mouth.

Are you now more convinced that oil pulling is right for you? There are still myths about it that you should know about. The next chapter will uncover it all.

Chapter 5: Common Misconceptions Of Oil Pulling

In a glance, oil pulling seems magical. This is what makes it easy for companies selling products and services to exaggerate their advertisements. Actually, it is really easy to believe things being said about oil pulling, most especially when many people have tried it and achieved desired results.

Your best defense against this tendency is to really know about the truths behind oil pulling. But wait, this book is all about this matter. As an alternative route, we will discuss about the common misconceptions about oil pulling. Through this, you will know what you shouldn't believe when you encounter people trying to sell products related to this procedure.

Consider the following:

- **Oil pulling is one of the newest health innovations available for us to make use of.** This is a misconception because this procedure has already been around a couple of centuries back. There are documents that could prove its use in Ayurvedic medicine that originated in India. The popularity of this procedure only caught on when bloggers started writing about it.
- **Only one type of oil can be used when doing this procedure.** This is actually misleading as a lot of oils can actually be used. If coconut, sesame, and sunflower oils are always being mentioned on published materials, this is because these are the ones easily available in many countries. Any oil which is organic, unrefined, and cold-pressed will be good for us to use.
- **Oil pulling can do whole body healing**. Actually, it is mainly focused on promoting the oral health of an individual. Since the mouth is connected to the digestive system which is in turn connected to other systems, getting its health up can be beneficial for the entire body in the long run. However, it is not right to think that it is an

automatic and direct cure to all illnesses that we might have.

- **Oil pulling can replace your dentist**. Again, this is wrong. Oil pulling can be used to enhance the health of your teeth and gums but it is never meant to replace your dentist. Yes, it can prevent the buildup of plaque or the development of tooth decay but proper dental services should never be ruled out of your list.
- **Toxins in the blood can be removed by oil pulling**. This is a misconception because oil pulling removes bacteria and microorganisms. Toxins that are in the body generally exist at the cellular level. If these are found on body cavities, such as the mouth, then we would have died a long time ago already. There is a slight chance that some nonlethal amounts of toxins are present in our mouth, but these will only bind to the oil being squished if they are fat-soluble.

There is no doubt that oil pulling really works when used as a natural form of oral care procedure. With its primary benefits leading to additional ones that many people have seen, there is no doubt that its popularity level will continue to rise in the days to come.

Are the benefits of oil pulling limited to oral health only? Turn to the next chapter for the answer!

Chapter 6: Other Benefits Of Oil Pulling

Yes, oil pulling can offer benefits that go beyond the aspect of promoting oral health. This is something that has been doubted before by a lot of the procedure's critics. Research results suggest that oil pulling will become more effective in the attainment of other health goals if it will be combined with good lifestyle practices and discipline. Of course, this is common sense. However, remember that the root of oil pulling is on Ayurvedic medicine, which takes into consideration principles of energy, nutrition balance, and mental health.

This means that even when it is logical that oil pulling clearly benefits the teeth, gums, and mouth, there are more benefits that you could expect out of it. These are enumerated below:

- **Keeps energy levels in check**: The body's system uses a lot of energy for its primary functions. When there is an increased abundance of microorganisms in the body, the immune system has to work much harder and this translates to the use of a whole lot more of energy. Since oil pulling leads to a decreased number of harmful microorganisms in the mouth, respiratory, and digestive systems, the immune system will not require additional amounts of energy.
- **Prevents hormonal imbalance**: Toxins and other chemical products of microorganisms can affect the production and presence of hormones. Oil pulling basically cuts off the source of these toxins and allows the body's endocrine system to function normally.
- **Leads to a more supple, smooth, and radiant skin**. By removing sources of toxins, the body's stress levels are also reduced. This promotes improved circulation of blood which is reflected on the quality of skin that you have. People who are practicing oil pulling procedures are observed to be better-looking and exhibit a more positive aura.
- **Acts as a migraine-suppressor**. The body has this mechanism of producing headaches or migraines when

there is a high level of stress or there's a need to recover. When toxins are removed through oil pulling, the existing migraine is suppressed or is decreased in severity.

- **Contributes to a restful sleep.** When the body's hormone, microorganism-induced stress, and toxicity levels are up, sleep patterns are detrimentally affected. The primary benefits of oil pulling leads to the normalization of these things. As a result, you will be able to attain normal patterns of restful sleep.

If you will notice, almost all of the additional benefits that you can get from oil pulling stems out from its ability to flush out the source of toxins: the microorganisms in the mouth. Oil pulling is definitely more than just a procedure to promote oral health. It is safe to call it a backup for the body's total health!

Chapter 7: How Oil Pulling Detoxifies And Cleanses

Contrary to the statements of those who doubt the detoxifying and cleansing benefits given by oil pulling, recent studies provide evidence for the power of this procedure or therapy. Yes, we can safely say now that oil pulling is a perfect way to detoxify and cleanse our body for better health. It appears that Ayurveda really has provided us with something that could solve our health concerns that begins at the mouth.

Now, let us examine closer how the process of detoxification through oil pulling happens. Basically, the body has this mechanism to dump toxins from the blood into the salivary glands. These biologically-generated toxins are fat-soluble which means they'll bind to a receptor or any substance that matches their molecular makeup. This is where the power of oil pulling is seen. Actually, the lipophilic reaction between the toxins and oils leads to the "pulling" action.

Saliva which contains these toxins is secreted out into the mouth. The toxins bind with the lipids found in the oil being squished around the teeth, gums, and whole mouth. The liquid that results that toxin-lipid binding makes the oil thin in consistency and this is an indication that the detoxification process has been successful. Through the help of the oil used in the process, your salivary gland becomes an organ of detoxification.

This explanation matches the data and findings on studies conducted in India, Australia, and US just a couple of months back. As for the cleansing power of oil pulling, its mechanics are easy to explain. We are actually referring to the cleansing of bacteria and other types of microorganisms that might be present in your mouth. The lipophilic principle that works in the detoxification process is also involved here.

The cell membrane of bacteria and other microorganisms are commonly made up of a fat-based compound. It means that if there is another substance with the same composition around, automatic binding will happen. In oil pulling, the cell membrane of bacteria gets attracted to the fats present on the oil. This makes them easy to flush out of the mouth.

Some types of oils have disinfecting properties which make them perfect as an alternative to mouthwash. True enough, oil pulling has been proven to give practitioners long-lasting fresh breath.

The detoxifying and cleansing power of oil pulling is definitely something that we shouldn't underestimate!

Chapter 8: Establishing An Oil Pulling Routine

The benefits and positive effects that oil pulling could offer cannot be yours after just a single session. There is a reason why this procedure is also referred to as a therapy. You have to do it consistently over a period of time. This means that you have to incorporate it into the daily routines that you have these days. This could be quite difficult, most especially if you are used to the fast-paced way of life today and exposed to conveniences such as commercially-available oral health products.

Of course, if you are really determined to get its benefits, learning and establishing an oil pulling routine is doable. The good thing is that in this chapter, you will learn about an oil pulling routine that still sticks to the traditional ways. Of course, the modern way of living has been put in consideration when this routine was designed.

Prepare in advance materials such as the following:

- Unrefined, cold-pressed, and organic sesame oil. If you don't have access to sesame oil, go for sunflower oil instead. Both of these have "warming energies" which are important in Ayurvedic medicine.
- A toothbrush which is going to be used only for the purpose of the oil pulling routine.
- Himalayan crystal salt. If this is not available, pick sea salt that is in its unrefined form.

Now that you have all the materials ready, it is time for you to establish the routine. Follow the steps presented below:

1. Just after getting out of bed in the morning, take a tablespoon of sesame oil and put it in your mouth. It is very important that you don't swallow it. Squish the oil around by using a combination of pulling and chomping motion. This isn't the same as gargling motion so it will really take

time for you to get used to it. Do this squishing for 20 minutes.

2. Spit out the oil which is supposed to have changed in consistency because of the presence of saliva and toxins pulled out from the mouth.

3. Mix salt and water into a drinking glass. Squish the mixture around your mouth. The purpose of this is to finally cleanse out the remaining toxins and oils that might have stayed behind.

4. Repeat if you desire so. If you will repeat process #1 to #3, make sure that your squishing motions are more aggressive.

5. Brush your teeth first with the oil pulling toothbrush and then with your regular toothbrush. You are free to use any toothpaste that you want. This last step is meant to finish off the cleansing process and to give you that fresh feeling that you are looking for.

Establishing this routine might be a little bit challenging, most especially if you have a very busy life. However, do it regularly and with the motivation to achieve a better level of oral health. There is a possibility that you'll pick it up as a habit in a shorter period of time.

Chapter 9: Best Techniques For Oil Pulling

After knowing about the basic steps in oil pulling, you are probably more confident about trying it. The entire process works as evidenced by many testimonials and research results published online. However, the degree of the positive results that you can possibly get will vary from those of others. Why does this happen? This is the same dilemma that also appeared when researchers tried the process on their respondents. It appeared that the results are affected by the technique that an individual will use when oil pulling.

Yes, there are techniques or advanced ways of doing the oil pulling routine. As the ancient Ayurvedic texts reveal, these are as follows:

- **Kavala technique**: In this technique, you will hold the sesame oil for a few minutes before starting the squishing motion. You will spit the liquid after 3 or 4 minutes. There is a need to repeat the entire procedure for 3 to 4 times if maximum positive results are desired.
- **Gandusa technique**: For this, you will have to hold the sesame oil longer in your mouth. A maximum time of 5 minutes is what needs to be allocated here. There will be no squishing. Just spit out the oil after the specified time. Of course, you will have to use more oil so that the gums and teeth will be covered. The process is repeated 2-3 times.

Because of many factors that could be present, there are variations on the kind of materials used for oil pulling. The condition of an individual's health and the desired results could be the determining points in deciding to mix up natural additives to the oil. Ayurvedic medicine texts have shown that even milk and honey could be added to the oil to achieve good results.

The use of specific oils in order to achieve certain results is recommended too. As an example, if fast cleaning and whitening of teeth is desired, you can use coconut oil which is known to have abrasive properties. Feel free to explore online information sources if you have specific needs or desires connected to the oil pulling routine you are planning.

While it is highly recommended that you do this oil pulling routine on mornings, there is really nothing wrong about doing it anytime you like. You can also repeat the process several times during the day if you want. Of course, be patient in waiting for the manifestation of positive results or outcomes. It could take days, weeks, or even months as explained on the previous chapters of this book.

Chapter 10: Things You Should Avoid While Oil Pulling

Oil pulling is definitely a very tempting thing to try these days. Its benefits are all there and there are no side effects to fear. The use of organic, unrefined, and cold-pressed materials also emphasizes further just how safe and beneficial oil pulling really is. However, this doesn't mean that there are no wrong ways of doing it.

If you are planning to establish your oil pulling routine soon, take note of the following things that you should avoid doing:

- *Gargling instead of squishing.* Squishing is much forceful and allows the oil to really come in contact with the teeth, gums, and all surfaces inside the mouth. Gargling for 10 to 20 minutes is also hard to do and can strain your mouth muscles.
- **Swallowing the oil.** This is actually the oil that you have squished around your mouth for 10 to 20 minutes. You are supposed to spit it out! The liquid is already full of bacteria and the toxins that have been pulled out of your salivary glands.
- **Aspiration of the oil.** Even if the oil is the "healthy" and naturally sourced, it can still harm your lungs. The worst case scenario is if you will aspirate the liquid which you are supposed to spit out. It will introduce pathogens into the lungs.
- **Replacing your brushing routine completely with oil pulling.** Remember that oil pulling alone cannot ensure the overall health of your mouth. As an example, plaque that has already accumulated cannot be removed by oil pulling. Brushing your teeth is included in the oil pulling routine as stated in the previous chapter. Don't forget to do it.
- **Using specific types of oil that you are allergic to**. There are many types of oil that can be used for the pulling routine. Do your research well or consult a medical professional if you really want to be sure on what to include in your oil pulling routine.

- **Not brushing one's teeth after oil pulling even after it has been included in the procedure.** The oil will coat the taste buds and will cause you to taste food differently. Of course, the bigger reason for you not to skip brushing is that there could still be a residue of the oil that contains toxins and bacteria present in the mouth. Even small amounts will lead to growth of bacteria and make the entire procedure useless.
- **Overdoing the process.** Remember to take things easy. Yes, it has been stated that you should do the oil pulling routine for 20 minutes. However, if you feel uncomfortable about doing it for the first time, do the next routine for a shorter period. Work your way up when you are finally getting the hang of it.

Now, there you have it all! Good luck on your oil pulling!

Conclusion

Thank you again for purchasing this book on *"Oil Pulling: Oil Pulling Beginner's Guide! - Learn How To Heal Your Body Using Nature's Ancient Detoxifying And Healing Oil Pulling Oral Detox Therapy Cleansing!"*

I am extremely excited to pass this information along to you, and I am so happy that you now have read and can hopefully implement these strategies going forward.

I hope this book was able to help you understand the seemingly complicated process of oil pulling and how to do the entire procedure according to traditional and modern principles mixed together.

The next step is to get started using this information and to hopefully live a happier and healthier life!

Please don't be someone who just reads this information and doesn't apply it, the strategies in this book will only benefit you if you use them!

If you know of anyone else that could benefit from the information presented here please inform them of this book.

Finally, if you enjoyed this book and feel it has added value to your life in any way, please take the time to share your thoughts and post a review on Amazon. It'd be greatly appreciated!

Thank you and good luck!

Ultimate Coconut Oil Guide!

<u>Coconut Oil</u>

Coconut Oil Recipes For Organic Skin Care And Natural Beauty, Clean Eating For Weight Loss, Shinning Hair, Better Brain Function And Overall Health!

Introduction

I want to thank you and congratulate you for purchasing the book, *Coconut Oil: Ultimate Coconut Oil Guide! - Coconut Oil Recipes For Organic Skin Care And Natural Beauty, Clean Eating For Weight Loss, Shining Hair, Better Brain Function And Overall Health!*

This book contains proven steps and strategies on how you can take full advantage of the beauty, weight loss and health benefits that coconut oil has to offer. Through this book, you will learn more about:

1. What makes coconut oil healthy?
2. How it can help you get better, more glowing skin.
3. Its effects on your hair and making healthier.
4. Can coconut oil improve your brain function?
5. Weight loss benefits and how it can boost your metabolism.
6. Coconut oil and how it can help treat different illnesses.
7. Recipes for both your diet as well as organic skin care.
8. How to choose the right coconut oil for your needs.

We hope that through this book, you'll be able to recognize the amount of potential that a single bottle of coconut oil contains.

Thanks again for purchasing this book, I hope you enjoy it!

Chapter 1: Coconut Oil For Natural Beauty And Health

These days, more and more people are becoming aware of the effects that chemically manufactured products has on their bodies. As such, many of them have turned to a greener, more organic lifestyle that advocates going all natural when it comes to their food as well as the different products that they use on their bodies.

This isn't surprising, of course, considering the fact that there are a number of illnesses which are associated with constant use of synthetic and often chemical-laden skin and health products. There are certain risks that one must bear when using it; risks which can be avoided altogether if one were to switch over to something that's a bit closer to nature.

The coconut oil is a favorite among health buffs as it is one of those by-products that can be used in a multitude of ways. On one hand, it can be eaten and taken as a supplement which would boost your overall health. On the other, it can be applied topically and used as a beauty product as well as a means of treating certain skin issues.

You get all of these benefits but without worrying about its harmful effects to the body.

Why is it considered one of the best natural remedies out there?

It's all in the composition. About 99% of it is composed of saturated fats (which, in this case isn't as bad as it sounds) as well as traces of polyunsaturated fatty acids and monosaturated fatty acids. Virgin coconut oil retains a higher amount of the good stuff thus it is also valued higher.

It also contains lauric acid and quite a generous amount of it at that. When digested by the body, this would turn into monolaurin and is very beneficial when it comes to dealing with different bacteria and viruses. Diseases such as influenza and herpes are just two of the things that coconut oil can cure in a jiff. A tablespoon of it a day keeps the doctor away, so to speak.

Besides these, it is also one of the most powerful inhibitors of quite a number of different pathogenic organisms ranging from your usual viruses to even protozoa. All of this, of course, is attributed to its high lauric acid content.

For beauty and skincare

Coconut can also be used for cosmetic or skin care purposes. We'll get to the specifics of this in later chapters but to quickly summarize, it is often used for: Hair care, skin care, nails, lips as well as treating different skin issues such as psoriasis. It helps keep the skin youthful and glowing as well as protect it from harmful UV rays.

Thanks for Previewing My Exciting Book Entitled:

"Coconut Oil: Coconut Oil Recipes For Organic Skin Care And Natural Beauty, Clean Eating For Weight Loss, Shinning Hair, Better Brain Function And Overall Health!"

To purchase this book, simply go to the Amazon Kindle store and simply search:

"COCONUT OIL"

Then just scroll down until you see my book. You will know it is mine because you will see my name "Sarah Brooks" underneath the title.

Alternatively, you can visit my author page on Amazon to see this book and other work I have done. Thanks so much, and please don't forget your free bonuses

DON'T LEAVE YET! - CHECK OUT YOUR FREE BONUSES BELOW!

Free Bonus Offer: Get Free Access To The www.LuxyLifeNaturals.com VIP Newsletter!

Once you enter your email address you will immediately get free access to this awesome newsletter!

But wait, right now if you join now for free you will also get free access to the "Secrets of Becoming A Meditation Expert – In 7 Days!" free Ebook!

To claim both your FREE VIP NEWSLETTER MEMBERSHIP and your FREE BONUS Ebook on the SECRETS OF BECOMING A MEDITATION EXPERT IN 7 DAYS!

Just Go To:

www.LuxyLifeNaturals.com

www.ingramcontent.com/pod-product-compliance
Lightning Source LLC
Chambersburg PA
CBHW061944280526
45787CB00004B/1721